Introduction and Summary

The Affordable Care Act (ACA) was passed against a backdrop of decades of rapid growth in health care spending in the United States. While much of this historical increase reflects the development of new treatments that have greatly improved health and well-being (Cutler 2004), there is widespread agreement that the system suffered from serious inefficiencies that increased costs and reduced the quality of care that patients receive. A key goal of the ACA was to begin wringing these inefficiencies out of the health care system, simultaneously reducing the growth of health care spending – and its burden on families, employers, and state and federal budgets – while increasing the quality of the care delivered.

This report analyzes recent trends in health care costs, the forces driving those trends, and their likely economic benefits. The report includes the following findings about recent trends:

- **Health care spending growth is the lowest on record.** According to the most recent projections, real per capita health care spending has grown at an estimated average annual rate of just 1.3 percent over the three years since 2010. This is the lowest rate on record for any three-year period and less than one-third the long-term historical average stretching back to 1965.

- **Health care price inflation is at its lowest rate in 50 years.** Recent years have also seen exceptionally slow growth in the growth of prices in the health care sector, in addition to total spending. Measured using personal consumption expenditure price indices, health care inflation is currently running at just 1 percent on a year-over-year basis, the lowest level since January 1962. (Health care inflation measured using the medical CPI is at levels not seen since September 1972.)

- **Recent slow growth in health care spending has substantially improved the long-term Federal budget outlook.** The Congressional Budget Office (CBO) has reduced its projections of future Medicare and Medicaid spending in 2020 by $147 billion (0.6 percent of GDP) since August 2010. This represents about a 10 percent reduction in projected spending on these programs. These revisions primarily reflect the recent slow growth in health care spending.

While the causes of the slowdown are not yet fully understood, the evidence available to date supports several conclusions about the slowdown and the role of the ACA:

- **The slowdown in health care cost growth is more than just an artifact of the 2007-2009 recession: something has changed.** The fact that the health cost slowdown has persisted so long even as the economy is recovering, the fact that it is reflected in health care prices – not just utilization or coverage, and the fact that it has also shown up in Medicare – which is more insulated from economic trends, all imply that the current slowdown is the result of more than just the recession and its aftermath. Rather, the

1

slowdown appears to reflect "structural" changes in the United States health care system, a conclusion consistent with a substantial body of recent research.

- **The ACA is contributing to the recent slow growth in health care prices and spending and is improving quality of care.** ACA provisions that reduce Medicare overpayments to private insurers and medical providers are contributing to the recent slow growth in health care prices and spending. In addition, ACA reforms that aim to improve the quality of care are reducing hospital readmission rates and increasing provider participation in payment models designed to promote high-quality, integrated care.

- **New economic research shows that the ACA's Medicare reforms are likely to reduce health care spending and improve quality system-wide.** Recent research implies that reforms to Medicare will have "spillover effects" that reduce costs and improve quality system-wide. In economic terms, this suggests that efforts to reform Medicare's payment system are "public goods."

- **Accounting for "spillovers" implies that the ACA's effect on health care price inflation may be much larger than previously understood.** The direct effect of ACA provisions that reduce Medicare overpayments to private insurers and medical providers has been to reduce health care price inflation by an estimated 0.2 percent per year since 2010. Accounting for the "spillover effects" discussed above raises this estimate to 0.5 percent per year, which represents a substantial fraction of the recent slowdown.

Slow growth in health care costs, thanks in part to the ACA, is likely to have substantial benefits for the Nation's economy in both the short-run and the long-run:

- **In the short run, slower growth in health spending is a positive for employment.** The slow growth in health care costs has reduced employers' benefit costs, increasing firms' incentives to hire additional workers. Available estimates suggest these gains could be substantial, although the magnitude is uncertain.

- **Over the long run, slower growth in health spending translates directly into higher wages and living standards.** If half the recent slowdown in spending can be sustained, health care spending a decade from now will be about $1,400 per person lower than if growth returned to its 2000-2007 trend, a benefit that workers will realize in the form of higher wages and that federal and state governments will realize as lower costs.

- **CBO estimates that the ACA will substantially reduce long-term deficits.** In large part because of the ACA's role in slowing the growth of health care spending, CBO estimates that the ACA will reduce deficits by about $100 billion over the coming decade and by an average of 0.5 percent of GDP ($83 billion per year in today's economy) over the following decade. These deficit savings are likely to grow over time and are separate from the revisions in CBO's Medicare and Medicaid spending projections that were discussed on the last page (which are not directly attributable to the ACA).

I.   Recent Trends in Health Care Costs

The first section of this report documents the historically slow growth in health care costs seen over the last three years. The main data used in this analysis are the most recent National Health Expenditures (NHE) Accounts projections, which were released by the Office of the Actuary at the Centers for Medicare and Medicaid Services (CMS) in September 2013 (Cuckler et al., 2013). These data are particularly well-suited to the task at hand, as they permit a detailed and comprehensive look at recent trends in the nation's health care spending.

It is important to note that the figures for 2012 and 2013 are CMS projections, although they are guided by actual data that are already available.[1] It is unlikely, however, that the final data will meaningfully change the conclusions below.[2]

Table 1 summarizes recent trends in spending growth, and Figure 1 depicts recent trends graphically. Over the three years since 2010, the real per capita annual growth rate of national health expenditures is just 1.3 percent, less than one-third of the long-term historical average growth rate of 4.5 percent and substantially below the average growth rates recorded from 2000-2007 and over the three years immediately prior.[3] The growth rate from 2010 to 2013 is, in fact, historically unprecedented. From the time this data series begins in the 1960s to the present, no earlier three-year period saw a lower growth rate.

The slow growth is reflected in all three payer categories, as also depicted in Figure 3, which appears on page 11. Real per enrollee spending growth in private insurance over the 2010-2013 period is approximately one-third its level from 2000-2007 and about one-half its level from 2007-2010. The effect on Medicare has been even more dramatic, with real growth in per beneficiary Medicare costs essentially ceasing over this period. In Medicaid, the already slow growth in real per beneficiary costs seen in recent years has given way to *reductions* in per beneficiary costs from 2010 to 2013.

The slowdown is similarly broad-based when looking across spending categories. Real per capita growth in spending on hospital care – the largest single category of spending, accounting for one-third of total spending – is growing at less than half the long-term historical average rate and more than 1 percentage point slower than the most recent historical period. Prescription drugs have seen particularly sharp reductions in growth, with spending actually shrinking in real per capita terms at a 1.6 percent annual rate over the last three years. Physician and clinical services and home health and skilled nursing care show similarly slow

---

[1] Specifically, CMS' methodology document indicates that these projections incorporate actual data on public health care programs extending through June 2013, and the document describes adjustments to the model output to better reflect actual data on private sector spending through 2012 (CMS Office of the Actuary, 2013a).

[2] In fact, on average in recent years, the CMS projections have actually modestly overstated health cost growth, and the typical forecast error in the growth rate has been 1 percentage point or less (CMS Office of the Actuary, 2013b). In addition, the basic trends portrayed by the CMS projections are similar to those seen in other data on health spending, which are discussed later in this section of the report.

[3] The periods 2000-2007 and 2007-2010 were chosen as comparison periods in order to facilitate the discussion in the next section of the role of the 2007-2009 recession in driving recent trends.

growth rates in a historical context, with the partial exception that the growth rate for physician and clinical services ticked up in 2010-2013 relative to the three years prior.

Table 1: Real per capita NHE annual growth rates, by payer and spending category

Category	Average annual growth rate, 2010-2013	Historical average annual growth		
		1965-2010	2000-2007	2007-2010
Total national health expenditures	1.3	4.5	3.9	1.8
Major payers (per enrollee)				
Private insurance	1.6	N/A	5.1	4.0
Medicare	0.0	N/A	5.4	2.3
Medicaid	-0.5	N/A	0.3	0.1
Major categories of spending				
Hospital care	1.9	4.3	3.9	3.2
Physician and clinical services	1.7	4.4	3.1	1.6
Prescription drugs	-1.6	4.7	6.2	0.3
Home health and skilled nursing care	1.1	6.5	2.9	2.7

Notes: The table reflects CEA calculations based on the CMS National Health Expenditures Accounts projections. Inflation adjustments were made using the GDP deflator. For consistency with the economic assumptions used in the CMS projections, calculations were made using the GDP deflator as reported by the Bureau of Economic Analysis before the comprehensive revisions in July 2013. Using the revised GDP deflator would have a negligible effect on the results. Per-enrollee growth figures are not available for the 1965-2010 period because Medicare and Medicaid did not exist in 1965 and because CMS does not provide enrollment data for private insurance (or any other insurance type) for years before 1987.

Figure 1

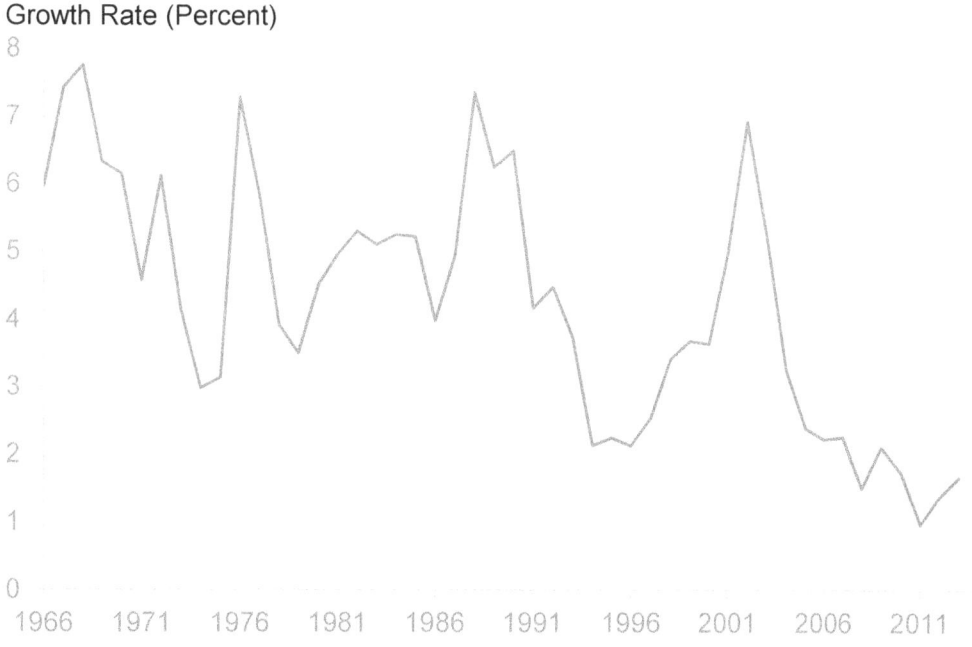

Real Per Capita Growth in National Health Expenditures

Growth Rate (Percent)

Notes: Figures for 2012 and 2013 are projections.
Sources: Centers for Medicare and Medicaid Services and Bureau of Economic Analysis.

The first half of Table 2 documents a similar slowdown in the *prices* paid for health care goods and services, which is also depicted in Figure 2. Health care inflation, whether measured using the personal consumption expenditure (PCE) price indices or the consumer price index (CPI) for medical care, is running at less than half the rate seen historically, and below the rates seen over the last decade. Indeed, in recent months, year-over-year inflation as measured using PCE data has been running at just 1 percent, a level last seen in January 1962. The recent behavior of the CPI for medical care is similar, with recent months' year-over-year inflation rates reaching low levels not seen since September 1972.

It is important to note that this slow growth in prices for health care goods and services is not simply a reflection of the fact that the prices of all goods and services have grown slowly in recent years. Panel B demonstrates that health care inflation *relative* to general price inflation has also been unusually low over the last few years.

Table 2: Recent trends in several indicators of health care spending and price growth

Category	Freq.	Avail. thru	Annual growth, ACA-present	Historical average annual growth		
				1965-ACA	2000-2007	2007-ACA
Panel A: Health care inflation						
PCE deflator, health care goods & services	Monthly	9/2013	1.8	5.7	3.3	2.8
CPI for medical care	Monthly	9/2013	3.1	6.3	4.3	3.5
Panel B: Health care inflation relative to general price inflation						
PCE deflator, health care goods & services	Monthly	9/2013	0.1	1.8	1.0	1.2
CPI for medical care	Monthly	9/2013	0.9	1.8	1.6	1.8
Panel C: Employer premiums (family coverage, adj. for inflation)						
KFF/HRET survey	Annual	2013	4.0	N/A	6.7	2.9
MEPS-IC	Annual	2012	3.6	N/A	6.3	3.2
Panel D: PCE on health care goods & services (adj. for inflation & pop.)	Monthly	9/2013	2.1	4.8	3.9	1.4

Notes: For monthly data, end points for periods starting or ending in a listed year are treated as occurring in July of that year. Employer premium growth is adjusted using the GDP deflator. Because MEPS-IC data are not available for 2007, the figures shown for that period reflect average growth rates for the period 2000-2006 and 2006-2010. For consistency with the NHE projections reported in Table 1, this table uses the GDP deflator as reported before the July 2013 NIPA revisions. PCE for health care goods and services includes the following categories of spending: health care, pharmaceutical and other medical products, therapeutic appliances and equipment, and net health insurance. This series is adjusted for inflation using the general PCE deflator and BEA's population series. The PCE deflator for health care goods and services includes the same PCE categories listed above; price indices for the constituent categories are combined to construct a Fisher index for the aggregate.

Figure 2

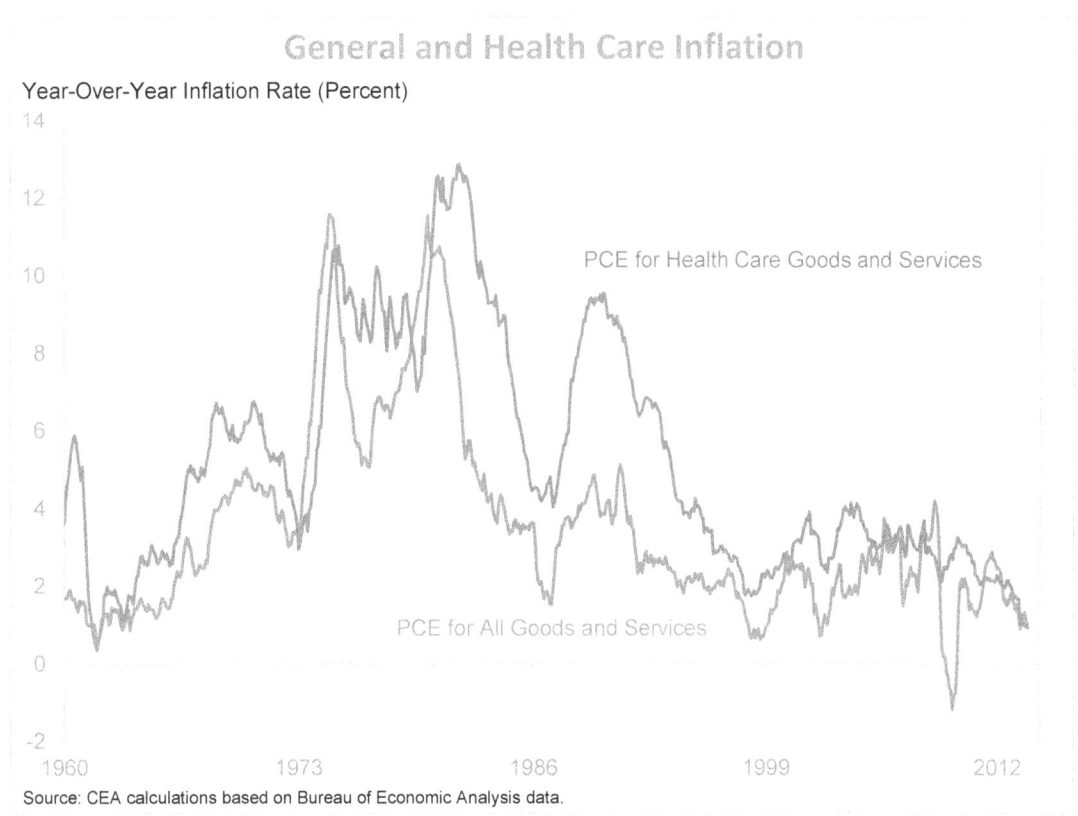

General and Health Care Inflation

Year-Over-Year Inflation Rate (Percent)

PCE for Health Care Goods and Services

PCE for All Goods and Services

Source: CEA calculations based on Bureau of Economic Analysis data.

Panel C of Table 2 examines trends in employer premiums, as documented in two major surveys of employers. In both surveys, premium growth rates are more than 2 percentage points below the 2000-2007 trend. Panel D tracks real per capita consumption spending for health care goods and services, based on data from the Bureau of Economic Analysis. By this measure, spending growth is running at about half the rate seen in the first portion of the last decade and even farther below its longer-term historical average. While these series do suggest that growth may have accelerated slightly since 2010, they are consistent with the other available data in showing that current growth rates are very low, whether measured against short-term or long-term historical experience.

This report examines two different measures of growth in health care costs: growth in the prices of health care goods and services and growth in total spending on health care goods and services. These two types of data are useful for answering different questions.

The growth in health care prices tells us how the amount of money needed to purchase a given amount of health care– a bypass surgery, a doctor's visit, or a tablet of aspirin – is changing over time. By contrast, the growth in health care spending captures not only changes in the prices of health care good or services (e.g. the price of a doctor's visit), but also changes in the quantity of health care goods and services consumed (e.g. the number of doctor's visits made).

Increases in health care prices (above general price growth) are unambiguously bad for households since they reduce the amount of health care a household can buy with a given number of (real) dollars. By contrast, increases in health care spending can be good or bad. If spending rises because households are receiving more care and that care improves health, then spending increases are a good thing. If, on the other hand, spending rises because the price of care is rising or because households are receiving additional care that does not improve health, then higher spending is a bad thing. Concern about the long-term growth in health care spending reflects a belief that much of that growth reflects higher prices or increased use of low-value care.

In practice, of course, measuring changes in health care prices is more challenging than in the idealized discussion presented above. In light of the rapid technological change that has been seen in the health care sector, it can be difficult to compare goods and services over time. For example, an appendectomy done in 1990 and an appendectomy done in 2010 might be treated as the "same item" in a health care price index, but it is likely that the 2010 version reflects substantial improvements in surgical technique relative to its 1990 counterpart, improvements that may be important for health outcomes. As a result, simply knowing that the price of an appendectomy has risen from 1990 to 2010 is not enough to determine whether someone in need of an appendectomy was better off in 1990 or in 2010.

Cutler et al. (1998) document that these measurement challenges are a substantial problem in practice. Focusing on care for heart attack patients, the authors show that mortality outcomes for these patients have improved dramatically in ways not accounted for in major price indices. As a result, these indices dramatically overstate the extent to which rising medical prices are making people worse off over time.

As a final note, to the degree that statistical agencies have gotten better at measuring quality improvements over time, long-term comparisons of health care price inflation can be misleading. Indeed, it is possible that some of the long-term decline in health care price inflation depicted in Figure 2 results from methodological improvements of this kind. However, methodological improvements of this kind are unlikely to play a substantial role over short time periods, and they likely play little or no role in explaining the sharp declines in health care price inflation over the last few years.

II. What is Happening Now, and What Will Happen Next?

A natural – and important – question is what is driving the recent slow growth in health care costs. The answer to this question can shed light on whether the current slow growth will last, and what policies could help make that occur. Indeed, slowdowns can be temporary; the early- and mid-1990s also saw several years of slow growth in health care costs, but costs accelerated once again in the late 1990s and early 2000s.

While final conclusions about the causes of the recent slow growth and its persistence await additional data and analysis, some conclusions are possible with the data currently available. Most importantly, the recent slow growth does not appear to be the result of idiosyncratic factors affecting a single category of spending or a particular payer. As documented in Table 1, the slowdown has affected all major payers and each of the major categories of spending. The search for explanations must, therefore, look for factors affecting behavior system-wide. The first part of this section examines the role of the 2007-2009 recession, the second part discusses potential non-ACA, non-recession explanations for the recent slow growth, and the third part considers the role of the Affordable Care Act so far and in the future.

The Role of the 2007-2009 Recession

Some have identified the 2007-2009 recession and its aftermath as a potential driver of system-wide changes. For example, jobs losses that led to reductions in insurance coverage could have reduced access to health care, or the accompanying reduction in families' disposable incomes could have led households to prioritize other needs over medical care. Alternatively, disruptions in financial markets could have depleted providers' cash reserves or reduced their ability to borrow in order to invest in new equipment or facilities, leading to lower utilization in subsequent years.[4] If the recession is the primary driver of the current slow growth in health spending, then health spending growth is likely to return to its earlier rapid rate as the economic recovery continues.

However, the theory that the slowdown in the growth of health care costs is simply a result of the recession is inconsistent with several pieces of evidence presented in Section 1.

- **The slowdown has persisted well beyond the end of the recession.** The Great Recession began in December 2007 and concluded by June 2009. Since that time, the economy has recorded four years of steady growth. Yet as shown in Table 1 and Figure 3, the growth rate of health spending has actually fallen further relative to the years during and immediately following the recession. While it is possible that the economy affects health spending with a lag, it seems likely that if the recession were the primary force driving the slowdown, some acceleration would be visible by now.

---

[4] The NHE data do show a very sharp reduction in investment in equipment and structures in the health care sector over 2009 and 2010 of about 13 percent in real per capita terms. It is worth noting, however, that this contraction followed two years of very strong investment growth. Moreover, even as financial conditions have normalized, investment has remained subdued, suggesting that providers do not view themselves as having incurred a substantial investment deficit, nor suggesting an imminent investment-driven rebound in health care cost growth.

- **The slowdown appears in Medicare, which is more insulated from the business cycle, not just the private sector.** One striking feature of the slowdown is that it has affected Medicare in addition to the private sector, a fact also documented in Table 1 and Figure 3. Because, in general, seniors are more insulated from a weak labor market, this fact undermines the notion the slowdown results primarily from income losses attributable to the recession. A recent analysis of recent Medicare trends by economists at CBO, which is discussed in greater detail below, lends additional credence to this view (Levine and Buntin, 2013). The director of CBO has indicated that this feature of the slowdown, along with its duration, is an important reason that CBO has sharply reduced its projections of future Medicare and Medicaid spending in recent years (Elmendorf, 2013).

- **The slowdown appears in health care prices in addition to health spending.** A final important piece of evidence is the recent dramatic slowdown in growth in health care prices, particularly the fact that health care inflation has slowed *relative* to inflation in the broader economy. These trends are documented in Table 2 and Figure 2. As discussed at the beginning of this subsection, there are a variety of plausible mechanisms by which the recession could reduce the quantity of health care services people demand and thus reduce total spending. By contrast, it is difficult to explain why a recession should cause a reduction in the growth rate of health care prices *relative to* price growth in other sectors of the economy. Thus, the recent behavior of health care inflation is difficult to square with the theory that the slowdown is primarily a result of the recession.

In addition, in recent months several different authors have rigorously evaluated the hypothesis that the recession is the primary factor driving recent slow growth in health care spending. These analyses, which use a variety of methods, have generally concluded that, while the recession likely has depressed health care spending growth in recent years, health spending is low in historical terms even after accounting for the recession. These results, together with the evidence catalogued above, suggest that a substantial portion of the recent slowdown is "structural," and thus is likely to persist. The remainder of this section provides a review of this growing literature.

Figure 3

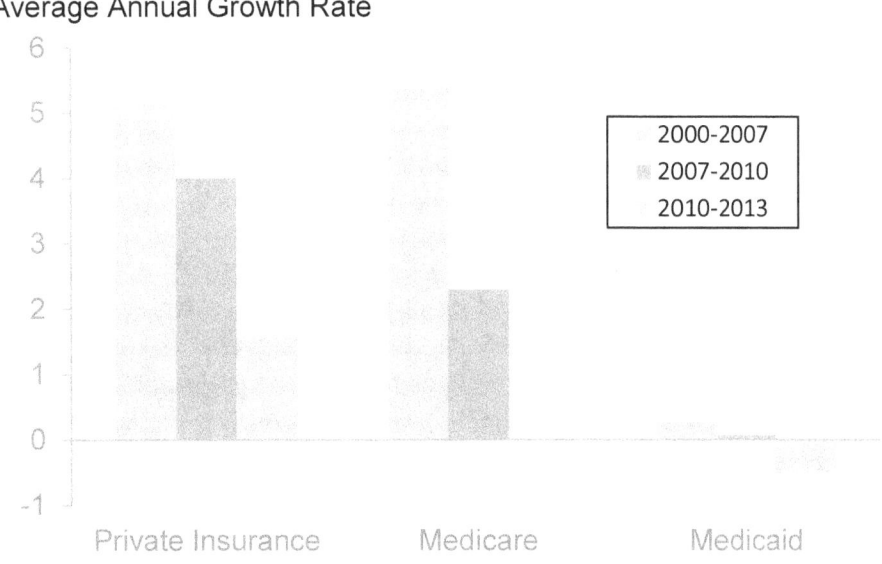

Real Per Enrollee Growth in Health Spending by Payer

Average Annual Growth Rate

Notes: Figures for 2012 and 2013 are projections.
Sources: Center for Medicare and Medicaid Services and Bureau of Economic Analysis.

One approach to evaluating the role of the recession is provided by Chandra, Holmes, and Skinner (2013). They survey the available micro-econometric estimates of the effect of income on the demand for health care. Virtually all such estimates in the existing literature are small, with the largest credible estimates of the income elasticity being the 0.7 estimate provided by Acemoglu et al. (forthcoming). Applying this upper-bound estimate to the observed slowdown in GDP growth, they show that the slow economic growth in recent years explains less than half of the recent slow growth in health spending. Although they express some uncertainty about the future outlook for health spending, they nevertheless project that a substantial fraction of the slowdown will persist, due in part to the potential of payment reforms included in the Affordable Care Act.

Another important piece of evidence on this comes from a recent analysis by economists at the Congressional Budget Office (Levine and Buntin, 2013). Levine and Buntin highlight the fact, discussed above, that the recent slow growth has appeared in Medicare as well as the private sector. Because, in general, seniors are more insulated from a weak labor market, this fact undermines the notion the slowdown results primarily from income losses attributable to the recession. In addition, Levine and Buntin find that, even to the extent seniors did experience economic disruption as a result of the recession, those experiencing relatively larger economic disruptions during the recession did not spend less on health care. Levine and Buntin also document, using state-level data on Medicare spending, that health spending growth has historically risen when unemployment rises, the opposite of the pattern required for the economic downturn to explain the slowdown in cost growth.[5]

Ryu et al. (2013) take another approach. They examine the role of two specific mechanisms by which the recession could have affected health care cost growth: reductions in insurance coverage due to job loss and increases in the cost-sharing faced by consumers due to firms' decisions to offer leaner health plans. Focusing on the period 2009-2011, they find that recent reductions in spending growth are, if anything, larger among employed individuals and that increases in cost-sharing can account for only one-fifth of the slowdown. On the basis of their results, they advise a "cautious optimism that the slowdown in health spending may persist."

Another set of studies evaluates the effect of the recession by estimating the historical relationship between economic growth and health spending growth and using this estimated relationship to simulate how health spending would have evolved had the recession not occurred. Econometric time series analyses like these have the important advantage that, by virtue of their nationwide, aggregate approach, they can capture the effects of a wide variety of potential mechanisms connecting economic growth to health spending growth. But the nationwide, aggregate nature of these analyses is also a weakness; it can be difficult to plausibly control for important confounding factors, and the paucity of data (only about 50 years of data, or about 50 total data points, are available) can make these analyses sensitive to seemingly innocuous changes in methodology, as demonstrated by Chandra, Holmes, and Skinner.[6] The current literature does not, unfortunately, provide persuasive evidence on which econometric specifications are likely to provide the most reliable results.

Cutler and Sahni (2013) estimate a model relating current health spending growth to a five-year average of economic growth. Based on their results, they estimate that spending growth in 2011 and 2012 would have been on the low end of the historical range even accounting for the recession, and that more than half of the slowdown over the longer period 2003-2012 is due to factors other than the recession. They conclude that "fundamental changes" are underway in the health sector, changes that are not attributable to the recession alone.

A contrary perspective comes from an analysis from the Kaiser Family Foundation and the Altarum Institute (KFF and Altarum, 2013). They estimate a model relating current health spending growth to economic growth in each of the last five years and general price inflation in each of the last three years. On the basis of these analyses, they conclude that most of recent slow growth in health care spending is attributable to the recession, although they still attribute 23 percent of the slowdown (over the longer period 2008-2012) to non-recession factors. It is

---

[5] The 2013 Economic Report of the President undertakes a related analysis (CEA, 2013). The report analyzes changes in state-level unemployment from 2007-2009 to state-level health spending growth over that period. While that analysis finds that unemployment does reduce health spending, the effect is small and cannot explain a substantial fraction of the recent downturn in health spending.

[6] Note that the CMS projections used in Section 1 also reflect the output of an econometric time series model and, thus, are subject to some of the same criticisms. However, as discussed in Section 1, CMS adjusts aspects of its 2012 and 2013 projections on the basis of actual data already available, so the shortcomings of the projection model are a substantially smaller concern in the present context.

important to note, however, that the authors' model, by virtue of its relative complexity, is particularly subject to the shortcomings of the time series approach that were described above. Indeed, the model estimated by KFF and Altarum has one particularly unusual feature: the effect of reduced economic growth on health spending actually peaks four years later. While not impossible, such lags seem implausibly long.

Other factors driving slower growth in health spending unrelated to the ACA

The recession does not provide a full, or even necessarily a major, explanation for the recent slow growth in health spending. What other non-ACA factors may be contributing to slow growth in recent years is still a subject of debate and research, but two have received substantial attention to date.

Increased cost-sharing may be reducing utilization in private plans

One factor that can plausibly explain why slow growth has affected many different categories of spending at the same time is a long-term trend toward increased patient cost-sharing (Cutler and Sahni, 2013; Ryu et al., 2013; Chandra, Holmes, and Skinner, 2013). The Kaiser Family Foundation/Health Research and Educational Trust Employer Health Benefits Survey indicates that recent increases in cost-sharing in employer plans have been substantial; the typical deductible in an employer plan has increased from $584 in 2006 to $1135 in 2013, a 70 percent increase after adjusting for inflation (KFF, 2013).

Some research suggests that the observed increase in cost-sharing is having an effect. As noted above, Ryu et al. (2013) examine the importance of increased cost-sharing in the employer context and conclude that it can account for 20 percent of the reduction in growth over the 2009-2011 period. Chandra, Holmes, and Skinner (2013) evaluate the role of increased cost-sharing using estimates from the literature of how utilization responds to cost-sharing. They conclude that cost-sharing may have played a larger role, although the precision of their estimates is limited by the poor quality of the available data on recent changes in cost-sharing and our incomplete understanding of how cost-sharing affects utilization.

As a final note, while it seems possible and perhaps likely that increased cost-sharing is playing a role, it cannot be the whole story. As discussed in detail above, the slowdown in Medicare fee-for-service spending has been even more dramatic than the slowdown in the private sector, and there have been no substantial changes to the core Medicare benefit design in recent years.

Many blockbuster drugs are coming off patent

Table 1 shows that the recent slowdown in prescription drug spending is particularly striking. A variety of sources attribute this sharp drop in prescription drug spending to the expiration of patent protection (or loss of market exclusivity) for many important drugs. Due to a slowdown in the invention of new drugs that dates back many years, these drugs are not being replaced by newly-invented drugs. As a result, the share of prescriptions accounted for by generic drugs has increased sharply, substantially reducing costs (Aitken, Berdnt, and Cutler, 2009; Cutler and Sahni, 2013; IMS, 2013). While these changes are almost certainly playing a role, it is important to note that their contribution to the aggregate trends is likely modest since prescription drugs account for less than 10 percent of total health spending.

The Role of the Affordable Care Act

A question of obvious interest, particularly in light of evidence that the recession is not the sole cause of the recent slow growth in health spending and that the other factors cannot explain the magnitude or broad scope of the slowdown, is the ACA's role in driving changes in the Nation's health care system. To be sure, the ACA is not the sole cause of the slowdown. Health care spending growth had slowed somewhat even before the ACA was passed (as shown in Section 1), the recession and other changes in the health system have certainly played contributing roles (as discussed above), and, in any case, many of the ACA's reforms are still coming online.

Nevertheless, the ACA's reforms aimed at driving out waste and improving quality are contributing to these trends in a meaningful way. Recent economic research also provides additional support for the premise that implementing reforms in Medicare can reduce the cost and improve the quality of care system-wide. This research confirms that the ACA will be critical to slowing health care cost growth going forward, but also suggests that its provider payment reforms may be having a larger-than-anticipated impact today.

Reductions in Medicare overpayments to providers and health plans

The ACA has already had one easily-quantifiable effect on the nation's health care spending: reducing overpayments previously identified by independent experts (e.g. MedPAC (2009)). The original Congressional Budget Office cost estimate for the ACA estimated that its reforms to Medicare would save $17 billion in fiscal year 2013, attributable primarily to reductions in payments to private insurers that provide coverage through Medicare Advantage and adjustments in annual updates to Medicare provider payment rates (CBO, 2010a).[7] Estimated savings of $17 billion constitute about 0.6 percent of national health expenditures in 2013. Spread out over the three years from 2010 to 2013, this implies that these effects of the ACA alone account for a 0.2 percentage point reduction in the growth of national health expenditures over this period, making a meaningful contribution to explaining the slow growth in health spending observed over this period. The analysis by Cutler and Sahni (2013) reaches similar conclusions.

Deployment of new payment models to increase efficiency and improve quality of care

The ACA also includes a wide variety of reforms intended to identify and diffuse models that promote efficient care delivery, reduce care fragmentation, and reward providers that invest in providing high-quality care, rather than just a high quantity of care.

The ACA made direct changes in Medicare payment models aimed at achieving these goals, including creating the readmissions reduction and shared savings programs discussed in detail below and various "value-based" purchasing initiatives that tie provider reimbursement to measures of the quality of the care received by patients. The Medicaid program has also made

---

[7] Elsewhere in this report, we cite a CBO estimate of the effect of the budgetary effects of repealing the ACA from July 2012. This estimate suggests that repeal would increase Medicare spending in FY2013 by $4 billion, a much smaller sum than the $17 billion cited here. However, as discussed in the CBO letter, because it would have been too late to unwind some ACA provisions for fiscal year 2013 and due to other effects, this estimate does not reflect the full effect in the ACA in that year.

available enhanced financial assistance to states that establish health homes to improve care management for patients with chronic conditions.

In addition, through the ACA-created Center for Medicare and Medicaid Innovation (the "Innovation Center"), CMS is experimenting with a wide variety of new payment approaches, including bundled payments, various accountable care models, and a variety of multi-payer initiatives discussed in the next section. Importantly, the Secretary of Health and Human Services will have the authority to take successful pilots to scale. To date, more than 50,000 health care providers from across every state are participating in an Innovation Center initiative.

Finally, through the Patient-Centered Outcomes Research Institute, the ACA is funding efforts to identify which treatments work – and for which patients – and to identify strategies for translating that evidence into practice. By giving providers the information they need to provide efficient, high-quality care, this important research initiative directly complements the ACA's efforts to change the incentives that providers face.

The remainder of this subsection discussed two ACA payment reforms that are well underway and are already beginning to show results:

- **Penalties for hospitals with high readmission rates:** One important change under the ACA is in how Medicare's hospital payment system treats hospital readmissions, cases in which a patient returns to the hospital soon after being discharged. Nearly one-in-five Medicare patients experienced such a readmission within 30 days as of 2010, and many of these readmissions are believed to result from low-quality care during the initial admission or poor planning for how the patient will obtain care after discharge. However, before the ACA, hospitals had no incentive to invest in activities aimed at reducing readmissions and could actually be made worse off by doing so since they would lose payment for the avoided readmissions. This misalignment of incentives likely both increased costs and reduced quality.

  The ACA corrects these incentives by penalizing hospitals with high readmission rates (among patients with a specified set of diagnoses). The rules governing these penalties were finalized in August 2011, took effect in October 2012, and will grow over time. Figure 4 provides evidence that this policy has begun changing patterns of care. After having been flat for several years, overall 30-day hospital readmission rates for Medicare patients turned sharply lower soon after the program rules were finalized, and are now nearly 1.5 percentage points below their average level from 2007-2011. While this decline may not be entirely attributable to the ACA payment incentives, these trends are encouraging (Gerhart et al., 2013).

Figure 4

Monthly Medicare 30-Day, All-Condition Hospital Readmission Rate
January 2007 - August 2013

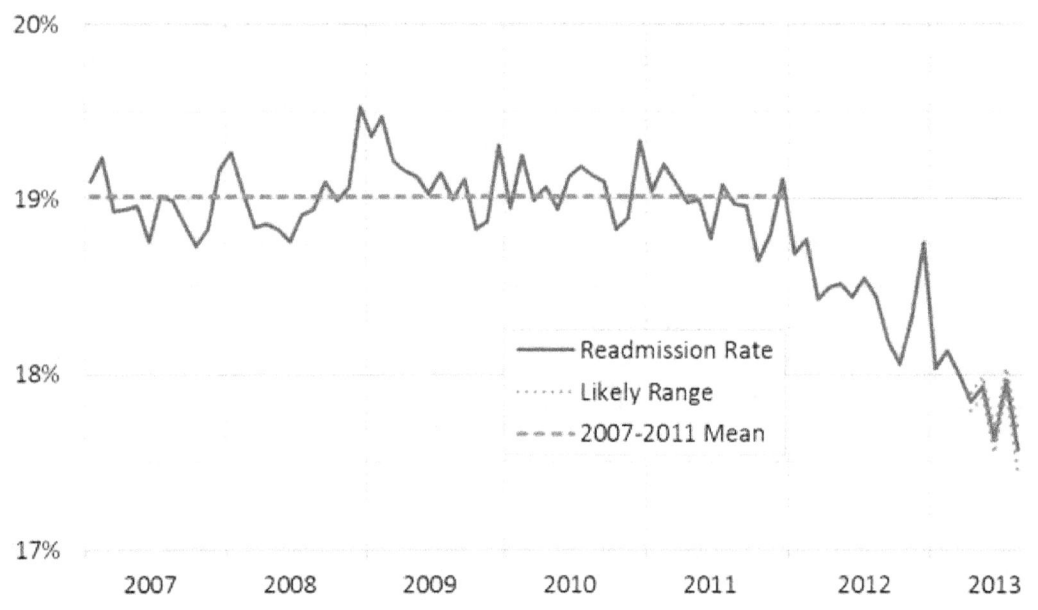

Source: Centers for Medicare and Medicaid Services, Offices of Enterprise Management.
Notes: A small number of claims for recent months have not yet been submitted. The estimates reported for recent months reflect the output of a CMS statistical model that accounts for this incomplete reporting. The dotted blue lines depict the range in which the final estimates are likely to fall once complete data are available, based on the output of the statistical model.

- **Accountable Care Organizations:** Another important ongoing reform under the ACA is the creation of "accountable care" payment models through the Medicare Shared Savings Program and the Innovation Center. These programs seek to realign provider incentives to encourage provision of efficient, high-quality care. Under fee-for-service payment systems, providers that find ways to provide more efficient care often end up financially worse off because lower service volume means lower payments from Medicare. In addition, since provider payments were based on service volume, the pre-ACA payment system gave providers no direct financial incentive to provide high-quality care.

  Under these programs, a provider or group of providers can seek designation as an Accountable Care Organization (ACO). ACOs are eligible to share in savings created when they increase the efficiency of the care for the patients they are responsible for. Because ACOs earn shared savings based on the total costs of a patient's care (across all providers) and not merely the costs for any particular visit or procedure, ACOs therefore have incentives to reduce care fragmentation and improve coordination. Perhaps most importantly, in order to be eligible for shared savings, ACOs must achieve designated benchmarks for the quality of care received by their patients, so ACOs have incentives to ensure that patients receive high-quality care.

Today, more than 240 organizations serving 4 million Medicare beneficiaries have adopted the ACO model, and it is likely that the number of beneficiaries covered will continue to grow in the years ahead. An initial CMS evaluation of the Pioneer ACO program (the Innovation Center ACO program for large and advanced systems) found that costs for beneficiaries aligned with Pioneer ACOs grew by just 0.3 percent in 2012, whereas costs for similar beneficiaries not aligned with ACOs grew by 0.8 percent. In addition, each ACO met or exceeded the program's quality benchmarks (CMS, 2013). While outside research on the effects of the ACO program itself is not yet available, research on similar private models suggests that they can achieve their intended purpose of reducing costs while improving quality (Song et al., 2012).

Research on cross-payer "spillovers" from Medicare to the private sector suggests that ACA's benefits may be larger than expected

In evaluating the direct effects of the ACA's Medicare and Medicaid reforms so far and considering their likely effects going forward, one important question is how these reforms will affect the rest of the health care system. Recent empirical work in economics and health policy strengthens the premise that reforms to public sector health programs that reduce waste and improve quality will have "spillover" effects on the private sector that generate savings and improve quality system-wide.[8]

In particular, a variety of recent studies suggest that efforts by Medicare to reduce excessive payments for particular services are likely to generate corresponding savings for private insurers and their enrollees. Clemens and Gottlieb (2013) study how the prices that private insurers pay to physicians change when Medicare changes its prices, exploiting a natural experiment created by regional differences in the effect of earlier reforms to the way Medicare pays physicians. They find that when Medicare reduces the price it pays for services, private insurers are able to reduce the amount they pay for care by similar amounts.

White (2013) and White and Wu (2013) undertake a similar analysis focused on Medicare payment to hospitals; they exploit natural experiments created by cross-hospital differences in the effect of earlier Medicare payment changes. White (2013) finds that when Medicare reduces its payment rates, private payers reduce their payment rates by approximately 77 percent of that amount. White and Wu (2013) find that for each dollar of Medicare savings, private insurers realize additional savings of 55 cents.

---

[8] This growing literature is contrary to the traditional view in some health policy circles which held that efforts to achieve savings in Medicare (or Medicaid) cause medical care providers to increase the prices they charge to private insurers in order to recover the lost revenue, and, thus, reforms in Medicare simply "shift" costs to the private sector rather than reducing them. The empirical support for this view was always inconsistent, and, as argued by Dranove (1988) and Morrissey (1994), this view has important conceptual shortcomings. In particular, for hospitals to be able to increase the prices charged to private payers after a reduction in Medicare payment rates, they must have been willingly charging a price below what the market would bear prior to the reduction in Medicare rates. For a comprehensive overview of this literature, particularly the older literature, see Frakt (2011; 2013).

The implications of these estimates are striking. Consider, for example, the estimated $17 billion in Medicare savings already achieved in fiscal year 2013 as a result of reducing Medicare overpayments. Applying the same logic applied previously, these estimated savings correspond to a 0.2 percentage point reduction in the average growth of health care *prices* over the period 2010-2013. If just half of these price reductions spilled over to the private sector to the extent estimated by White (2013), then the implied reduction in health care inflation economy-wide due to these Medicare changes would be about 0.5 percent. In this scenario, the ACA would be playing a significant role in driving the observed slow growth in health care prices—representing about one-half of the recent slowdown in health care inflation relative to general price inflation.[9]

Potentially even more important, the work by Clemens and Gottlieb provides evidence that the benefits of the ACA's improvements to the *structure* of public sector payment systems may be realized system-wide, not just among enrollees of those programs. Again focusing on Medicare payment for physician services, they show that Medicare payment changes that increase payment for some services and reduce payment for others tend to be matched by private insurers. Clemens and Gottlieb's results provide empirical support for the widely-believed notion that Medicare's payment structure serves as the "starting point" in negotiations between providers and private insurers, in which case changes in Medicare will reasonably quickly get picked up in the private sector as well. This evidence is consistent with historical experience. Medicare introduced "prospective" payment in the 1980s, under which all care during an inpatient admission was covered via a single payment determined based on the patient's diagnosis; virtually all private insurers pay hospitals using this type of system today.

Some recent evidence suggests that spillover benefits from the ACA's public sector payment reforms may arise even if private payers do not directly adopt these payment models. McWilliams et al. (2013) study the Alternative Quality Contract, an ACO-like contract that Blue Cross Blue Shield of Massachusetts has been experimenting with since 2009. Research cited above (Song et al., 2012) finds that the AQC reduces costs and improves quality for patients whose care is directly subject to the contract. The research by McWilliams et al. finds, however, that patients associated with AQC-participating providers whose care was *not* subject to the contract (in this case, Medicare patients) also experienced improvements. In this case, the cost savings amounted to 3.4 percent, on average, and these cost savings arose alongside improvement on some quality measures. The results may arise because providers adopt a single "practice style" for all their patients, so that practice style changes induced by one payer have effects on all patients.

Taken together, the evidence of cross-payer spillovers reviewed above suggests that not only are reforms to the structure of the public sector payment systems helpful in reducing costs and improving quality system-wide, but that the public sector may be *essential* to such

---

[9] Of course, effect on total spending may be smaller or larger to the extent that these price changes induce changes in volume. Indeed, the estimates of White and Wu, referenced above, as well as estimates reported by He and Mellor (2012) suggest that volume changes will generally work to offset these price spillovers. However, even under the estimates of White and Wu (2013), the savings to private insurers as a result of Medicare changes would be substantial.

improvements. In economic terms, the presence of spillovers means that payment system reforms are classic "public goods," investments that generate benefits for many people other than the purchaser and for which the purchaser cannot capture all the resulting benefits (Clemens and Gottlieb, 2013). Because no individual investor captures the full benefits of investment in public goods, the private market generates too few of them. As with other public goods, one solution to the underinvestment is for the government to invest directly, in this case by implementing reforms itself through Medicare and Medicaid.

Recognizing the importance of the decisions of other payers in determining the response of providers to new payment arrangements, CMS has launched demonstration projects that actively engage multiple payers. By incorporating multiple payers into reform efforts at the outset, these activities may increase the possibility that the payment models that emerge can easily cross payer boundaries once proven. These initiatives also recognize that engaging private payers in reform efforts is important for Medicare and Medicaid beneficiaries *themselves*, in light of the evidence described above that spillovers can run in both directions: from Medicare and Medicaid to the private sector, but also vice versa.

HOW WILL THE ACA'S COVERAGE EXPANSION AFFECT TOTAL SPENDING GROWTH?

Recent projections suggest that, as the ACA's coverage expansion comes online, health care spending may grow at an elevated rate for a few years, reflecting the cost of covering an additional 25 million people (Cuckler et al., 2013; CBO, 2013a). This one-time increase in costs is more than justified by the benefits of bringing quality, affordable health insurance coverage to millions of Americans who do not have it today. It should be neither a surprise, nor a cause for concern.

It is also worth noting that the projected increase in growth is not particularly large. Even after accounting for transient effects attributable to the ACA's coverage expansion, CMS projects that annual real per capita growth in national health expenditures will never exceed 3.4 percent over the next decade. As shown in Table 1, these rates are below the average growth rate recorded over the period 2000-2007 and far below the longer-term historical average.

Regardless, this one-time change will tell us nothing about the underlying trend in health spending, and it is underlying trend that, as discussed in Section 3, will shape Americans' living standards over the long run. Similarly, the experience over the next few years will not provide an accurate reflection of the ACA's long-term impact on the growth of health care spending. The ACA's Medicare reforms are slated to continue to phase in over years beyond 2014, and the ACA's mechanisms for generating new innovative reforms aimed at reducing costs and improving quality are just beginning to generate results. As a result, the savings from these and other aspects of the ACA are likely to grow substantially over time. This is an important reason why the Congressional Budget Office estimates that the extent to which the ACA will reduce the deficit grows dramatically over time (CBO, 2012b).

Two multi-payer initiatives merit special mention. Through the Comprehensive Primary Care Initiative, CMS has enlisted public and private payers in seven states to join with Medicare to invest in primary care practices, with the goal of getting those practices ready to participate in a shared savings model within two years. Another promising effort is the State Innovation Models Initiative, which provides grants to states that wish to make statewide, multi-payer changes to provider payment systems. With support from this program, Oregon has embarked upon an effort to move its Medicaid participants, state employees, and Marketplace enrollees into ACO-like payment models. Arkansas has undertaken an initiative involving public and private payers aimed at ensuring that half of Arkansans have access to a patient-centered medical home by 2016 and expanding its existing system of episode-based payment.

III.   Economic Benefits of Slow Health Spending Growth

Slower growth in health care costs has the potential to bring with it three important economic benefits: lower deficits, potentially generating faster economic growth; higher living standards; and, at least in the short-run, higher employment. This section of the report considers the implications of slower growth in health care cost along all of these dimensions.

Lower deficits and faster economic growth

In 2012, the Federal government devoted 22 percent of its budget, or 4.6 percent of GDP, to Medicare and Medicaid. For this reason, the future path of growth for health care costs has major implications for the long-term budget outlook.

Over the last three years, the Congressional Budget Office (CBO) has made a series of downward revisions to its forecast of future spending on Medicare and Medicaid (CBO, 2010; 2011; 2012c; 2013a), which are depicted in Figure 5. From the projections CBO published in August 2010 to its most recent set of projections in May 2013, CBO has reduced its estimate of Medicare and Medicaid spending in 2020 (the latest year covered by all of the projections examined here) by $147 billion or 0.6 percent of GDP. This represents about a 10 percent reduction in spending on these programs.

These reductions primarily reflect lower projections of future growth in health care costs.[10] To that point, in a recent presentation, CBO director Doug Elmendorf commented, "The slowdown in health care cost growth has been sufficiently broad and persistent to persuade us to make significant downward revisions to our projections of federal health care spending" (Elmendorf, 2013).

---

[10] There was one significant change in CBO's projections during this period that reflected factors other than changes in CBO's expectations about the growth of health care costs: the June 2012 Supreme Court decision in NFIB v. Sebelius. CBO materials indicate that this ruling reduced projected Medicaid spending in 2020 by roughly $30 billion as of July 2012, although this figure has likely fluctuated somewhat as CBO has changed its assumptions about how many states will adopt the Medicaid expansion. For a more detailed discussion, see CBO's analysis of the budgetary effects of the Supreme Court decision (CBO, 2012c) and CBO's March 2012 baseline (CBO, 2012a).

For comparison, in CBO's most recent long-term budget outlook, CBO projected that the current law 25-year fiscal gap – a measure of the annual fiscal adjustment required to stabilize the debt as a share of the economy over the next 25 years – is just 0.9 percent of GDP (CBO, 2013b). Without these recent improvements in the outlook for federal health spending, the nation's fiscal problem would therefore be more than half again as large.

Figure 5

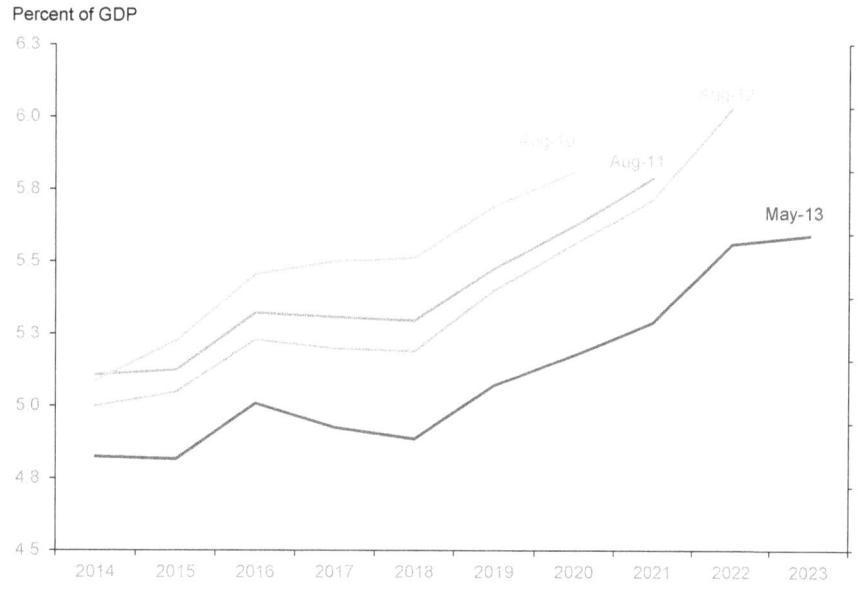

Recent CBO Projections of Medicare and Medicaid Outlays

Source: Congressional Budget Office projections.
Notes: Medicare outlays reflect spending net of offsetting receipts. Figures for the May 2013 projections reflect CBO's initially published projections, which did not account for recent NIPA revisions.

These reductions in long-term deficits have the potential to improve economic growth. Reductions in long-term deficits increase national saving, which increases capital accumulation and reduces foreign borrowing, and thereby national income and living standards over time. As discussed in detail in a 2009 CEA report on the potential benefits of health care reform for the economy, this means that even modest sustained reductions in health care cost growth can generate substantial economic benefits (CEA, 2009).

It is important to note that the reductions in projected Medicare and Medicaid spending described above are separate from the deficit reduction that CBO estimates will occur as a direct result of the ACA. The most recent CBO estimates indicate that the ACA will reduce the deficit by about $100 billion over the decade 2013-2022, and that it will reduce the deficit, on average, by about 0.5 percent of GDP in the subsequent decade (CBO, 2012b). CBO expects these deficit reducing effects will continue to grow thereafter.

Higher living standards

All else equal, when the health sector consumes less of the Nation's output, more resources are left over for meeting other needs. As a result, reductions in health care spending that arise from improving efficiency or eliminating low-value care have the potential to improve living standards. Because of the large share of the Nation's resources devoted to health care, even relatively modest percentage reductions can have very large effects on economic well-being.

PREMIUMS ON THE ACA MARKETPLACES ARE LOWER THAN PROJECTED

Recent research has found that premiums on the ACA Marketplaces are 16 percent below the level derived from earlier Congressional Budget Office estimates (ASPE, 2013). This has two important benefits. First, lower premiums will result in lower Federal costs for premium tax credits and cost-sharing assistance (Spiro and Gruber, 2013). Second, lower premiums will mean lower costs for many families, including those with incomes too high to qualify for premium tax credits and those that wish to purchase more comprehensive coverage than that offered by the second-lowest cost silver plan.

While the reasons that premiums on the ACA Marketplaces are lower than expected are not yet fully understood, this may be another benefit of the slow growth in health care spending documented in this report. The Marketplaces may also have proved better than expected at encouraging insurers to compete on price (Spiro and Gruber, 2013). A related possibility is that the Marketplaces attracted greater-than-expected participation by insurers; premiums appear to be substantially lower in areas with more participating insurers (ASPE, 2013).

These benefits accrue to families through two channels. First, standard economics implies that, in the long run, since employers must compete for workers, reductions in the cost of providing health benefits are passed through to workers in the form of higher wages (Summers, 1989). This theoretical prediction has received empirical support (Gruber and Krueger, 1991; Gruber, 1994; Baicker and Chandra, 2006). Second, as discussed in detail above, lower health care costs have significant benefits for the Federal budget, which ultimately permit lower taxes or increased investment in other valued public services.

One straightforward way of illustrating the magnitude of the potential impacts is to consider the effect of continuing the slow growth of the last few years. To that end, recall from Table 1 that national health expenditures have grown at a 1.3 percent real per capita annual rate from 2010-2013, whereas they grew at a 3.9 percent rate from 2000-2007. Suppose that half of that slowdown continued, so that instead of returning to the recent historical rate of 3.9 percent, real per capita health care costs instead grew at a 2.6 percent rate, similar to the rate projected in the recent work by Chandra, Holmes and Skinner (2013). Under this illustrative scenario, the savings after a decade would amount to about $1400 per person. As discussed above, these savings would materialize in the form of higher wages and lower state and federal costs.

Higher employment

Slower growth in health care costs reduces the growth of the health insurance premiums paid by employers. As discussed above, because employers must compete for workers, reductions in the cost of health care are likely to be passed through to workers in the form of higher wages in the long run. Thus, over the long run, changes in the growth rate of health care costs are unlikely to substantially affect employer's hiring costs and hiring decisions.[11]

In the short run, however, the picture may differ. Wage setting is subject to various "rigidities" that mean that lower health insurance costs may not be fully passed through in the short and medium run, potentially reducing employer costs and spurring hiring (Sommers, 2005). Rigidities of this kind may be particularly important in the aftermath of the 2007-2009 recession, as abnormally low inflation has increased the importance of constraints on the adjustment of nominal wages (Daly et al., 2012).

There is relatively little empirical literature on the effect of slower growth in employer health insurance premiums on employment, and there is no consensus among economists about the likely size of these effects. There are, however, at least two empirical studies suggesting that these effects could be substantial.

Baicker and Chandra (2006) use variation in employer health insurance costs resulting from within-state changes in medical malpractice costs over time to estimate the effect of higher health insurance premiums on employment. They find that a 10 percentage point reduction in employer premiums increases the share of working-age individuals who are employed by 1.2 percentage points. This estimate suggests that the recent slowdown in the growth of health insurance premiums could have had a substantial effect on employment.

Sood, Ghosh, and Escarce (2009) take an alternative approach to quantifying the effect of faster premium growth on employment. Specifically, they examine whether industries that provide insurance to a large share of their employees experience relatively lower employment growth during periods when health costs are growing particularly rapidly. They find that, for an industry that provides health insurance to all of its workers, increasing health insurance premiums by 1 percentage point reduces the industry's employment growth by 1.6 percentage points relative to an industry that insures none of its workers.

Translating the Sood, Ghosh, and Escarce estimates into effects on aggregate employment is difficult because their results could arise either because higher health insurance costs reduce employment overall or because they cause a reallocation of employment from high-insurance industries to low-insurance industries. Cutler and Sood (2010) make plausible assumptions about the importance of these two types of employment changes, and given their estimates of

---

[11] Faster growth in health insurance costs could reduce employment through another mechanism. In particular, if workers do not value the additional health spending, then the combination of more expensive health insurance and lower wages could make employment less attractive over time, inducing them to reduce their labor supply. Because evidence suggests that workers' labor supply is only modestly responsive to the returns to work, these effects are likely to be modest in size.

the effect of the ACA on the path of health care costs, find that the ACA will increase job growth by 250,000 to 400,000 per year by the second half of this decade.

IV. Conclusion

The evidence is clear that recent trends in health care spending and price growth reflect, at least in part, ongoing structural changes in the health care sector. The slowdown may be raising employment today, and, if continued, will substantially raise living standards in the years ahead. The evidence also suggests that the ACA is already contributing to lower spending and price growth and that these effects will grow in the years ahead, bringing lower cost, higher quality care to Medicare and Medicaid beneficiaries and to the health system as a whole. But realizing these benefits will require additional action, including continuing aggressive implementation of the ACA's reforms, taking full advantage of the ACA's mechanisms for developing and deploying innovative new payment models, and pressing forward with new efforts that build on the ACA's approach to reducing health spending system-wide, like the reform proposals in the President's fiscal year 2014 budget.

References

Aitken, Murray, Ernst R. Berndt, and David M. Cutler. "Prescription Drug Spending Trends in the United States: Looking Beyond the Turning Point," *Health Affairs*, 2009, 28(1), 151-160.

Assistant Secretary for Planning and Evaluation, Office of. "Health Insurance Marketplace Premiums for 2014," 2013, http://aspe.hhs.gov/health/reports/2013/MarketplacePremiums/ib_marketplace_premiums.cfm.

Baicker, Katherine and Amitabh Chandra. "The Labor Market Effects of Rising Health Insurance Premiums," *Journal of Labor Economics*, 2006, 24(3), 609-634.

Chandra, Amitabh, Jonathan Holmes, and Jonathan Skinner, "Is This Time Different? The Slowdown in Healthcare Spending," Brookings Panel on Economic Activity, September 2013, http://www.brookings.edu/~/media/Projects/BPEA/Fall%202013/2013b%20chandra%20healthcare%20spending.pdf.

Centers for Medicare and Medicaid Services Office of the Actuary. "Accuracy Analysis of the Short-Term (11-Year) National Health Expenditure Projections," 2013, http://www.cms.gov/Research-Statistics-Data-and-Systems/Statistics-Trends-and-Reports/NationalHealthExpendData/downloads/ProjectionAccuracy.pdf.

Centers for Medicare and Medicaid Services. "Pioneer Accountable Care Organizations succeed in improving care, lowering costs," 2013, http://www.cms.gov/Newsroom/MediaReleaseDatabase/Press-Releases/2013-Press-Releases-Items/2013-07-16.html.

Centers for Medicare and Medicaid Services Office of the Actuary. "Projections of National Health Expenditures: Methodology and Model Specification," 2013, 1-31.

Clemens, Jeffrey and Joshua D. Gottlieb. "Bargaining in the Shadow of a Giant: Medicare's Influence on Private Payment Systems," National Bureau of Economic Research Working Paper, 19503, 2013, 1-64.

Congressional Budget Office. "Cost Estimate of H.R. 4872, Reconciliation Act of 2010 (Final Health Care Legislation)," March 2010, http://www.cbo.gov/publication/21351.

Congressional Budget Office. "The Budget and Economic Outlook: An Update," August 2010, http://www.cbo.gov/publication/21670.

Congressional Budget Office. "The Budget and Economic Outlook: An Update," August 2011, http://www.cbo.gov/publication/41586.

Congressional Budget Office. "Updated Budget Projections: Fiscal Years 2012 to 2022," March 2012, http://www.cbo.gov/publication/43119.

Congressional Budget Office. "Letter to the Honorable John Boehner providing an estimate for H.R. 6079, the Repeal of Obamacare Act," July 2012, http://www.cbo.gov/publication/43471.

Congressional Budget Office. "Estimates for the Insurance Coverage Provisions of the Affordable Care Act Updated for the Recent Supreme Court Decision," July 2012, http://www.cbo.gov/sites/default/files/cbofiles/attachments/43472-07-24-2012-CoverageEstimates.pdf.

Congressional Budget Office. "An Update to the Budget and Economic Outlook: Fiscal Years 2012 to 2022," August 2012, http://www.cbo.gov/publication/43539.

Congressional Budget Office. "Updated Budget Projections: Fiscal Years 2013 to 2023," May 2013, http://www.cbo.gov/publication/44172.

Congressional Budget Office. "The 2013 Long-Term Budget Outlook," September 2013 http://www.cbo.gov/publication/44521.

Council of Economic Advisers. "The Economic Case for Health Care Reform," 2009, http://www.whitehouse.gov/assets/documents/CEA_Health_Care_Report.pdf.

Council of Economic Advisers. "Economic Report of the President," 2013, http://www.whitehouse.gov/administration/eop/cea/economic-report-of-the-President/2013.

Cuckler, Gigi A., Andrea M. Sisko, Sean P. Keehan, Sheila D. Smith, Andrew J. Madison, John A. Poisal, Christian J. Wolfe, Joseph M. Lizonitz and Devin A. Stone. "National Health Expenditure Projections, 2012-22: Slow Growth Until Coverage Expands And Economy Improves," *Health Affairs*, 2013, 32(10), 1-12.

Cutler, David. 2004. *Your Money or Your Life: Strong Medicine for America's Health Care System*. New York, NY: Oxford University.

Cutler, David and Neeraj Sood. "New Jobs Through Better Health Care: Health Care Reform Could Boost Employment by 250,000 to 400,000 a Year this Decade," *Center for American Progress,* 2010, http://www.americanprogress.org/issues/2010/01/pdf/health_care_jobs.pdf.

Cutler, David and Nikhil R. Sahni. "If Slow Rate of Health Care Spending Growth Persists, Projections May Be Off by $770 Billion," *Health Affairs*, 2013, 32(5), 841-850.

Daly, Mary, Bart Hobijn, and Brian Lucking. "Why Has Wage Growth Stayed Strong?" *FRBSF Economic Letter*, 2012, 1-10.

Dranove, David. "Pricing by Non-Profit Institutions," *Journal of Health Economics*, 1988, 47-57.

Elmendorf, Doug. "The Slowdown in Health Care Spending," Brookings Panel on Economic Activity, September 2013, http://www.cbo.gov/publication/44596.

Acemoglu, Daron, Amy Finkelstein, and Matthew J. Notowidigdo. "Income and Health Spending: Evidence from Oil Price Shocks," *Review of Economics and Statistics*, forthcoming.

Frakt, Austin B. "The End of Hospital Cost Shifting and the Quest for Hospital Productivity," *Health Services Research*, 2013, 1-10.

Frakt, B. Austin. "How Much Do Hospitals Cost Shift? A Review of the Evidence," *The Milbank Quarterly*, 2011, 89(1), 90-130.

Gerhardt, Geoffrey, Alshadye Yemane, Peter Hickman, Allison Oelschlaeger, Eric Rollins, and Niall Brennnan. "Medicare Readmission Rates Showed Meaningful Decline in 2012," *Medicare & Medicaid Research Review*, 2013, 3(2), E1-E12.

Gruber, Jonathan. "The Incidence of Mandated Maternity Benefits," *American Economic Review*, 1994, 84(3), 622-641.

Gruber, Jonathan and Alan B. Krueger. "The Incidence of Mandated Employer-Provided Insurance: Lessons From Workers' Compensation Insurance," *Tax Policy and the Economy*, 1991, 5, 111-143.

He, Daifeng and Jennifer M. Mellor. "Hospital volume responses to Medicare's Outpatient Prospective Payment System: Evidence from Florida, *Journal of Health Economics*, 2012, 730-743.

IMS Institute for Healthcare Informatics. "Declining Medicine Use and Costs: For Better or Worse?," 2013.

Kaiser Family Foundation. "2013 Employer Health Benefits Survey," 2013, http://kff.org/private-insurance/report/2013-employer-health-benefits/.

Kaiser Family Foundation and Altarum Institute. "Assessing the Effects of the Economy on the Recent Slowdown in Health Spending," 2013, http://kff.org/health-costs/issue-brief/assessing-the-effects-of-the-economy-on-the-recent-slowdown-in-health-spending-2/.

Levine, Michael and Melinda Buntin. "Why Has Growth in Spending for Fee-for-Service Medicare Slowed?," Congressional Budget Office, Working Paper, 2013-06, 2013.

McClellan, Mark, David M. Cutler, Joseph P. Newhouse, and Dahlia Remler. "Are Medical Prices Declining? Evidence from Heart Attack Treatments," *The Quarterly Journal of Economics*, 1998, 113(4), 991-1024.

McWilliams, J. Michael, Bruce Landon, Michael E. Chernew. "Changes in Health Care Spending and Quality for Medicare Beneficiaries Associated With a Commercial ACO Contract," *Journal of the American Medical Association*, 2013, 310(8), 829-836.

Medicare Payment Advisory Commission. "Improving Incentives in the Medicare Program," 2009, http://www.medpac.gov/documents/jun09_entirereport.pdf.

Morrissey, Michael A. *Cost Shifting in Health Care: Separating Evidence from Rhetoric*, 1994, Washington DC: American Enterprise Institute.

Ryu, Alexander J., Teresa B. Gibson, M. Richard McKellar, and Michael E. Chernew. "The Slowdown in Health Care Spending in 2009-11 Reflected Factors Other than the Weak Economy and Thus May Persist," *Health Affairs*, 2013, 32(5), 835-840.

Sisko, Andrea, Christopher Truffer, Sheila Smith, Sean Keehan, Jonathan Cylus, John A. Poisal, M. Kent Clemens, and Joseph Lizonitz. "Health Spending Projections Through 2018: Recession Effects Add Uncertainty to the Outlook," *Health Affairs*, 2009, 28(2), 346-357.

Sood, Neeraj, Arkadipta Ghosh and Jose J. Escarce. "Costs, Use and Outcomes: Employer-Sponsored Insurance, Health Care Cost Growth, and the Economic Performance of U.S. Industries," *Health Services Research*, 2009, 1-16.

Sommers, Benjamin D. "Who Really Pays for Health Insurance? The Incidence of Employer-Provided Health Insurance with Sticky Nominal Wages," 2005, 5, 89-118.

Song, Zirui, Dana Gelb Safran, Bruce E. Landon, Mary Beth Landrum, Yulei He, Robert E. Mechanic, Matthew P. Day, and Michael E. Chernew. "The 'Alternative Quality Contract,' Based on a Global Budget, Lowered Medical Spending and Improved Quality," *Health Affairs*, 2012, 31, no.8, 1885-1894.

Spiro, Topher and Jonathan Gruber. "The Affordable Care Act's Lower-Than-Projected Premiums Will Save $190 billion," 2013, http://www.americanprogress.org/issues/healthcare/report/2013/10/23/77537/the-affordable-care-acts-lower-than-projected-premiums-will-save-190-billion/.

Summers, Lawrence H. "Some Simple Economics of Mandated Benefits," *The American Economic Review*, 1989, 79(2), 177-183.

White, Chapin. "Contrary To Cost-Shift Theory, Lower Medicare Hospital Payment rates For Inpatient Care Lead To Lower Private Payment Rates," *Health Affairs*, 2013, 32(5), 935-943.

White, Chapin and Vivian Yaling Wu. "How Do Hospitals Cope with Sustained Slow Growth in Medicare Prices?," *Health Services Research*, 2013, 1-21.